Belly Dancing and Beating the Odds

Belly Dancing and Beating the Odds

How one woman's passion helped
her overcome breast cancer

Yvette Cowles

Harper
TrueLife

HarperTrueLife
An imprint of HarperCollins*Publishers*
77–85 Fulham Palace Road,
Hammersmith, London W6 8JB

www.harpertrue.com
www.harpercollins.co.uk

First published by HarperTrueLife 2014

1 3 5 7 9 10 8 6 4 2

© Yvette Cowles 2014

Yvette Cowles asserts the moral right to
be identified as the author of this work

A catalogue record of this book is
available from the British Library

ISBN: 978-0-00-810511-2

Printed and bound in Great Britain by
RR Donnelley at Glasgow, UK

I would like to dedicate this book:

To anyone whose life has been touched by cancer;

*To all my belly dancing buddies for their laughter,
friendship and inspiration;*

*And, of course, to my mother, Mrs Doreen Cowles,
'my rock', without whom none of this would have
been possible.*

'When it rains it pours. Maybe the art of life is to convert tough times to great experiences; we can choose to hate the rain or dance in it.'

Joan Marques

Chapter 1

The Seeds of an Obsession

Little did I know when I first discovered belly dance that it would turn into a life-long obsession, take me to far-flung places, provide me with the best friends I could ever wish for and keep me going through some of the darkest periods of my life. My first encounter with belly dance took place in the exotic surroundings of St Étienne, a town in eastern France best known for coal mining, bicycles and a moderately successful football team.

My love affair began while I was round at Samira's house, enjoying mint tea and cake with the girls. Samira had put on some Arabic music and Naget picked up a hip-scarf and started to dance to it. Her hips shimmied so vigorously that the coins rattled and the fringing flew. While she danced the rest of the girls clapped and ululated – a sound known as the *zaghreet* – enthusiastically. It was captivating.

So it was that I discovered my passion for Arabic music and dance. At that time I was 22 and teaching English as a language student in a multicultural secondary school in St Étienne. My colleagues were pleasant enough but quite reserved, and I was quite perturbed when one of them gave me a signed picture of Jean-Marie Le Pen, president of the Front National, as a welcome present. I was lonely and homesick, but Samira, Naget and the other North African girls in my class took me under their wing, invited me round to their houses for mint tea and welcomed me into their world.

When Naget finished dancing she handed *me* the scarf. I was petrified! My legs turned to jelly, I was rooted to the spot and my hips wouldn't budge. But, little by little, thanks to the warmth and encourage-ment of my new-found sisters, I learned to shed my inhibitions, let go and enjoy myself. My hips happily made the circles and 'figure eights' that the girls taught me, and my shoulders shimmied as enthusi-astically as theirs. After years of stressing about my weight, and struggling with anorexia and bulimia, at last I had discovered a sensual and mesmerising dance form that celebrated the female form and could look beautiful whatever a woman's age, size or shape. I was completely entranced.

Those afternoon dance sessions became a regular fixture. I loved those girls and their families; they made me feel that I belonged. And I saw belly dance as an expression of that sisterhood and sharing. For them it was just something that women did when they got together. But then they didn't know the white middle-class London suburbs where I was brought up! By the time I left France I was desperate to stay but the academic year was over, my contract was finished and I had to go back to Exeter to complete my degree. And there were no belly dancers there. So the sparkly scarf that the girls had given me as a leaving present was put in a drawer, where I almost forgot about it.

After leaving university I hadn't a clue what to do next so gave in to my mother's persistent pestering to do a secretarial course. How I hated it! But thanks to my newly acquired secretarial skills – and the fact that my star sign was compatible with that of my new manager – I got my first job: Promotions Assistant with a well-known London publisher.

It was 1987 and part of my job – pre-Internet – was to scour the papers for reviews of books by our authors. One day, as I was flicking through the *Sunday Times*, a headline caught my eye: 'Belly Dance Classes for Health and Relaxation'. They were being run by Tina Hobin at Pineapple Dance Studios, just around the corner from the office! So began the second chapter of my dance story …

I dusted off the hip-scarf, started going to regular classes, and immediately became hooked. And I wasn't alone. I had fallen among fellow addicts who, like me, just couldn't get enough of the intoxicating music, sensual dancing – and the dressing up, of course! The more we danced and studied, the more we realised how much there was to learn, so we went to as many classes and workshops as we could to improve our technique and extend our repertoire.

We started practising our shimmies and hip-drops at each others' houses, sharing cassettes of Arabic music with each other, and eagerly devouring clips of the stars of Egyptian dance on VHS – video cassettes copied so many times that the picture was grainy and the dancer barely distinguishable. But it didn't matter; we loved what we could see, and those stars, Samia Gamal, Tahia Carioca and Fifi Abdou, became our idols.

A friend asked me to dance at her father's birthday party, which had an Arabian Nights theme.

'Oh no, I'm just a beginner,' I protested, 'I'm really not good enough.'

'But Yvette, you'll be great,' Sarah pleaded. 'Just dance for a bit and then get everyone to join in. It is Dad's fiftieth, after all. There must be some consolation for being that old!' I had to agree that 50 was pretty ancient, so how could I refuse?

I enlisted my mother to help me make a costume. Before she got married, she had been a seamstress with a London couture house and had been constantly in demand from friends and family to create dresses for weddings, christenings and other special occasions. She would make the off-cuts into stylish creations for me and I would dance around my bedroom, wafting chiffon scarves and spinning as fast as I could to make my skirts swirl. My dressing-up box was legendary in my school. And, thanks to Mum, I acquired a life-long passion for silk, chiffon and other fine fabrics. No drip-dry crimplene for me! Although my mother was completely bemused by my passion for belly dance and viewed sequins and spangles as rather 'vulgar' and 'showy', between us we came up with an eye-catching pink two-piece (known in Arabic as a *bedlah*). The bra and hip-belt took me weeks to decorate with jewels and swathes of bugle bead fringing and, when combined with nine yards of chiffon skirt that floated and swirled as I danced, the result was a labour of love that made me feel like a princess.

The night of the party didn't start well. I was so anxious that I got lost, drove the wrong way down a one-way street and nearly collided with a van. Thinking that the other driver was going to get out and punch me, I reversed at speed, driving my car into a large oak tree. When I arrived, Sarah's house was much bigger than I expected; and there were dozens of cars outside. So much for the 'small, intimate gathering' Sarah had promised me! By the time I plucked up the courage to ring the door-bell I was in quite a state. My hairpiece had dislodged, my make-up was halfway down my face, I'd lost one earring and I looked wild-eyed and slightly unhinged. The look on Sarah's face as she opened the door spoke volumes. The sea of Aladdins, sultans and harem girls parted for me and I dashed upstairs to a bedroom to repair the damage.

Half-an-hour later I emerged, make-up and dignity restored, enveloped in a gold and pink sequined veil. I walked downstairs with all the enthusiasm of a woman about to face a firing squad. I'd given Sarah a tape of the music; I just prayed it would work. And that my costume would remain intact; in rehearsal the day before my bra strap had come unhooked as I practised my shoulder shimmies. The assembled friends and family were all sitting in the 'large reception room', the size of a barn. There was a magician on just before me and I could hear the laughter and chorus of 'Abracadabra' two floors up in the bedroom. Oh well, I thought, at least everyone seems to be in a party mood.

As I waited in the hall for the strains of *Aziza*, my entrance music, I felt a sharp twinge in the pit of my stomach. My hands were shaking so much that I kept dropping my veil. I thought of the legendary Fifi Abdou, one of the stars of Egyptian dance, and my greatest inspiration. What would *Fifi* do? It was obvious; she would command the stage and have the audience hanging on her every hip-drop. A hush descended. I took a deep breath and made my grand entrance.

The next 15 minutes are something of a blur. I just remember snatches – the smiling faces, roars of appreciation and applause, plus the pure, unadulterated pleasure that I experienced. Every fibre of my being tingled with energy; I had never felt so alive! I shimmied and sashayed around the room, twirling and spinning with my veil, before draping it over the astonished birthday boy and coaxing him to dance with me. By the end of the second track the whole room were on their feet and I was teaching them to *zaghreet* – the high-pitched sound of appreciation that Naget and the girls had taught me – and camel walk across the floor. I finally made my exit to a chorus of cheers, and remained in a euphoric daze for several days afterwards. A delighted Sarah told me that my first solo gig had been 'a triumph!'

My first performance had been such an intoxicating experience that I was soon hungry for another fix. My new-found sisters and I formed a group and started dancing at school fêtes, retirement homes, shopping centres – basically, anywhere that would have us. We didn't mind the wet and windy weather, the filthy dance floors, the less than salubrious changing conditions, or even the leery men – we were girls together having a great time! I felt the same sense of sisterhood and sharing that I had with my North African friends.

I had always loved dancing. As a child I went to ballet classes but I had a 'sticky-out bottom' and didn't fit in. I tried ballroom dancing but felt desperately self-conscious being 'in hold' –

especially with boys! I liked to put on my favourite pop songs and dance freestyle, choreographing little routines and imagining myself catching the eye of the cameramen on *Top of the Pops*. That all changed when I reached adolescence, a miserable period that brought exams, stress, self-loathing and the onset of anorexia. Instead of dancing around my bedroom, I cocooned myself in it all day, writing poems about death. Happily, in France my passion for dance had been re-ignited, and better still, I had found a dance style that really suited me. Not only did I love the music, the costumes and the fact that I was continuing a strong female tradition, but my body enjoyed the movements – at times sinuous, at others percussive – and took to them quite naturally. And once I had acquired a repertoire of movements, I could put them together to express the music as I really felt it.

Through our teacher, Tina, I met a group of other professional dancers and formed an association, MEDA-UK, designed to promote belly dance and give dancers an opportunity to meet up and share information about classes, performances and other activities. For some reason, I was made chairperson. I was only 24 and the least experienced dancer there, but the consensus was that if I worked in publishing I must be quite intelligent, well organised and therefore up to the job. I did tell them that my current responsibilities didn't extend much beyond filing and tea-making, but it didn't seem to matter. Or maybe, unlike me, they knew what I was letting myself in for; at times managing such big personalities really put my diplomatic skills to the test. But that certainly proved very handy in later years when dealing with some of my more temperamental authors!

One of MEDA-UK's biggest achievements was our charity fundraising. Ironically – given how much support I would receive from them myself in later years – one of the most successful events was a fundraiser at Chelsea Harbour for the Royal Marsden Hospital. But the ones I am most proud of are the Belly Dance-Ins that we ran for three years in the Covent Garden Piazza. Without the benefits of emails and social media, we gathered together over 100 dancers from all over the country, had great fun and raised lots of money for charity. Two of our leading members, Vashti and Jill Chartell, pulled strings, called in favours and got big names involved with amazing media coverage. Our friends and families rallied round and even my rather bemused parents weren't safe – they got roped in to selling Turkish delight, my dad in a rather fetching *galabeya* and *fez*. It was a magical time.

I started going to other classes and eventually started classes of my own, where I could share my passion for the dance and encourage others to find theirs too. Many of the women came out of curiosity; some of them were businesswomen, some mothers eager for a break from the kids and a night out with their friends, some of them were looking for a form of exercise that was a little more exciting than keep-fit, others were inspired by dancers they'd seen on their holidays to Egypt or Turkey. A number were very lacking in confidence and obviously very self-conscious. I knew that feeling! They arrived in baggy t-shirts and leggings and looked askance when I asked them if they would like to borrow a hip-scarf. But a few weeks later they were fighting each other for the most sparkly and jangly one to wear.

And so my dance and publishing careers carried on in parallel. They each fulfilled a different need in me. I loved working in publishing because it was such a creative environment and I learned something new from every author and colleague that I worked with. I was given more and more responsibility and bigger campaigns to work on. I loved the challenge. It enriched my mind every single day. But belly dancing was the antidote to all that – I felt it reconnected me with my body and nourished my soul. Whatever their merits, both lives were all-consuming and, what with classes, rehearsals, shows and publishing conferences and launch parties, left little time for anything else. My biggest problem was that there were only 24 hours in the day, and I did need a handful of them for sleeping. Even being in a relationship didn't deter me. 'I'm very low down the pecking order, aren't I?' sighed my boyfriend, as I went off to yet another dance weekend somewhere around the country. I felt a pang of guilt, but it didn't stop me. There was so much to do, and I was determined not to miss out on any of it.

Chapter 2

Cancer - Round One!

I was leading a charmed life – and then in 1996 my luck ran out. While I was showering one day, I felt a lump. I went to the local Well Woman clinic and they thought it was a *fibroadenoma*, commonly known as a 'breast mouse'. The doctor assured me that there was no real cause for concern, but given that my mother had had breast cancer, she referred me to the Royal Marsden Hospital to be checked out anyway. At that time the Breast Diagnostic Unit was housed in a portacabin.

'Has it been here long?' I asked the receptionist.

'Twenty-five years,' she replied.

I had the breast biopsy and blood tests, but again nobody seemed very concerned. And then, I received a call from one of the nurses, asking me to come back as there had been a mix-up with the tests and they needed to re-do them. My boyfriend offered to come with me but in the circumstances I couldn't see the point. It was only a few tests. When I went back and was shown into the consulting room, I took off my top and waited for the consultant to appear. He looked puzzled when he came into the room.

'Why have you got undressed?'

'Because you're re-doing the tests, aren't you?' He looked rather awkward.

'We really don't need to. We already know the results. And I'm afraid you have DCIS, or *ductal carcinoma in situ*. It's the earliest possible form of breast cancer.'

I could barely register what he was saying. I had genuinely believed the nurse, but it had merely been a ruse to get me back without causing me undue alarm. Cancer. The very word made me shudder. And I'd supported my mother through breast cancer four years before and was only too aware of what she'd been through. But she had been 60 and I was only 31. The consultant went on to say that, although DCIS isn't a life-threatening condition, if left untreated it may develop the ability to spread into the surrounding tissue and become an invasive breast cancer. For that reason I would need a lumpectomy and then, once the cells had been examined, we would discuss further options such as radiotherapy and hormone treatment.

After the appointment I called my mother, my boyfriend and a couple of close friends. I thought that by telling them it would feel more real, but I was still numbed by the news. That evening I was due to drive up with a colleague to a sales conference in Market Bosworth. In spite of my mother's misgivings, I decided to go. I had to keep busy and not have too much time to think. Ironically though, one of the titles being presented was a book on breast cancer. During the presentation the editor reeled off a handful of statistics. 'One in nine women will get breast cancer in their lifetime' was one; '80 per cent of women who develop breast cancer are over 50' was another.

I was devastated. 'Why me, and why so young?' I asked myself. I didn't know anyone my age with cancer. Besides, I just didn't have time to be ill. I had loads of deadlines coming up at work, not to mention a dance show and classes to prepare for. A few days after being diagnosed, I went to see the surgeon at the Royal Marsden Hospital, who told me that I would have to come in for surgery the following week. My boyfriend looked on in horror as I told the surgeon in no uncertain terms that it would be impossible as my assistant was going to be on holiday. The surgeon shook his head, ignored my protests and I was admitted a few days later.

I was really anxious about being disfigured. Before the operation, the surgeon marked the area to be removed with a black marker pen. It looked like a sizeable chunk to me. 'Do you really need to take away *that* much?' I asked him. Apparently they did. I came back from surgery heavily bandaged up and the nurses were sensitive to my concerns, only removing them when I felt ready to see the scars. There was a noticeable dent but it wasn't so bad; I had prepared myself for worse.

It was a small ward and my fellow patients were lovely. They were different ages and at different stages of their treatment, but we all supported each other. I also had an endless stream of visitors, including my belly dance buddies. They transformed my drab little cubicle into a sequined boudoir and bought a flurry of much-needed fun and colour. Their antics really cheered me up – not to mention the rest of the ward. My close friend and dance partner, Margaret, even turned up one day carrying a huge black bin-liner, with a pink plastic arm protruding from it. With great glee she removed an inflatable man – complete with a strategically placed banana and a pair of her three-year-old's underpants. We nicknamed him Dick Rogers and he became the ward mascot, moving from one bed to another as they became vacant during the course of the week. In fact, by the time I left, the nurses had become so attached to him that I thought it only fair to leave him in their capable hands.

During my operation the surgeons had removed some lymph nodes under my arm, to see if the cancer had spread. Thankfully, they were all clear. We then had to decide on the course of follow-up treatment. Because the cancer had been at such an early stage, there were several options open to me: radiotherapy, tamoxifen – an anti-oestrogen drug – both of the above, or neither. I opted for both, as I wanted to give myself the best possible chance of ensuring that the cancer didn't come back.

Radiotherapy was a daily business. The treatment itself lasted only a few minutes but the whole procedure could take ages if you had to wait, or if, as happened sometimes, the equipment broke down. I was lucky that I worked in Hammersmith and could commute to work afterwards. It was fine at first, but I did get progressively more tired as the course went on. But my manager and the rest of the team were very supportive. I even managed the odd dance class, although I just went through the paces and had to be careful with my arm.

I was just grateful that the cancer had been caught at a very early stage and that I'd got away without a mastectomy and chemotherapy. I was also immensely relieved that I was being treated at the Royal Marsden. I knew I was in safe hands there, and getting the best care that the NHS could provide. And I supplemented all the medical treatment with a course in acupuncture and some spiritual healing. I felt tired and rather fragile, but listening to Arabic music and choreographing new dances in my head, plus the support and camaraderie that I got from my students and fellow dancers, really got me through a difficult time and made me determined to get better so I could perform again.

Just as importantly, the dancing helped me recon-
nect with my body. Like a number of women I've
spoken to, I couldn't help feeling that my body had
let me down. How dare it do this to me! My complex
about my weight, my generous bottom and other
perceived defaults, was now compounded by
concerns about the big dent in my breast and the
ugly scar in my armpit. But allowing myself to enjoy
the flowing and sensuous movements made me feel
better about myself; it was a relief to know that I
could still feel womanly.

Once I'd been through the treatment, I tried to
put the whole cancer episode behind me. I was still
taking tamoxifen, but other than that, I just needed
to attend regular check-ups and have an annual
mammogram. The consultant said that there was a
25–40 per cent chance of the cancer coming back,
but I preferred to ignore those statistics. Back then
there wasn't a great deal of support for younger
women with breast cancer and my circumstances
were different from those of the older women I'd
met. Rather than dwell on what I saw as an unfortunate 'blip', I wanted to move on and get on with my
life. Up to that point, I'd felt invincible; no matter
how much I punished my body, it always bounced
back. I had to hope that this time would be no
different.

Chapter 3

Escape to France

My dancing and publishing careers both went from strength to strength. I was promoted to Non-Fiction Marketing Director and enjoyed all the kudos that went with it – the big campaigns, the launch parties, working with some of the biggest names in publishing. Every day was different, with new challenges and new experiences; I never knew what to expect. I loved my job and couldn't have been happier.

At the same time I was pursuing my love of dance. I taught regular classes at Jacksons Lane in North London and organised shows and parties for my students. I hosted workshops for international teachers and I went to courses with top dancers in Paris, Berlin, New York and San Francisco. I met some fantastic women and inspirational dancers – my network of belly dance buddies had gone global!

Over the years I have been to Egypt many times, but it was my first visit to Cairo, irresistible to any belly dancer, that made an indelible impression on me. I went on a trip organised by a work colleague, whose father was general manager of the Cairo Sheraton Hotel. From the moment the plane touched down, I was dazzled: the smells, the noise, the colours and the vibrancy of the city, that some in our party found quite overwhelming, were all magical to me. One evening, a member of our party suggested that we went to a belly dance show at the hotel's night club, as the dancer-in-residence was apparently 'Egypt's biggest star'. After the meal a seemingly endless succession of singers, folkloric dancers and entertainers took to the stage. Then, at 3am, the dancer appeared. It was Fifi Abdou herself! She was older and considerably less svelte than on the grainy videos I had seen of her, but even more compelling in the flesh; the archetypal *maalima* or boss woman, with a relaxed yet commanding style – and the best shimmy in the business.

For the next two hours Fifi danced, entertained, sang, smoked a *shisha* pipe and told jokes, through a variety of costume changes, from a startling purple and yellow *bedlah* to a fitted *baladi* dress to the man's traditional *galabeya* she wore to perform the *raqs el tahtib* or men's stick dance. There were undoubtedly more elegant and refined dancers, but none with her energy, exuberance and sheer *joie de vivre*. I idolised her for her dancing, and for dragging herself up from poverty to become not just Egypt's best-paid belly dancer, but the richest woman in Egypt. Fifi had dealt with a number of obstacles along the way;

the fundamentalists who regularly denounced her and the 'morality police' who decided that her movements were so lewd that they threw her into jail more than once. Undaunted by such setbacks, she continued to do what she loved most. What a woman! I would have been happy with an ounce of her nerve and courage.

I returned from Egypt even more inspired. I longed to perform on a proper stage, with professional sound and lighting, and a captive audience. Then, as so often has happened, the opportunity presented itself. I was invited to join Josephine Wise's Masriat Dance Company as a soloist, and to be involved in my first theatrical show. Thanks to Jo, I even had the opportunity to perform in an opera, Bizet's *Djamileh* at the Linbury Studio of the Royal Opera House. And not many belly dancers can claim that!

Very few of my gigs were that glamorous. But even the grotty ones make me smile to look back on. I – and my boyfriends over the years – were never keen on cabaret or restaurant work, but I did sometimes cover for friends at gigs when they were double-booked or needed time off. It wasn't my natural habitat; publishing is a female-friendly industry, and I was used to being treated with a degree of respect. Here, I found that some of the managers and waiters were patronising and sexist. They would 'accidentally' walk in on you while you

were changing in the cupboard they had thought-
fully provided and make you hang around for hours
before you got paid. I also hated the enthusiasm with
which some men tried to stick money down my
costume and even found myself backing off when
they approached with a note (rather foolish given
how little I was being paid). But I did enjoy getting
people up to dance, particularly the women.
I remember one New Year's Eve in Grayshott
dancing on tables and then leading a conga around
the village green, while the restaurant kept my
boyfriend happy by giving him a slap-up meal and
unlimited drinks.

Probably the most bizarre experience was a book-
ing three of us went to on a cold winter night in a
Turkish restaurant in Reading, located directly
opposite a cemetery. When we arrived, the place was
packed out with Hells Angels. It was nine o'clock
and already there were women throwing up in the
toilets. 'Are you sure about this?' I asked Margaret,
who had been liaising with the restaurant. 'Oh yes.
It'll be fine,' she assured me. Hmm, I thought, I've
heard that before.

When the women started spitting and warning us
not to make a move on their men – something that
most certainly was not about to happen – I felt a
sense of impending doom. We danced and the
response was enthusiastic, but not at all welcome.
'You're better than strippers,' one said. 'If we pay

you more, will you take your tops off?' said another. I was most affronted. 'Belly dancing is *not* stripping. It's an art form, you know!' I protested, but they just laughed.

I was ready to leave until we hit on the idea of putting on some Black Sabbath instead of our usual Arabic repertoire. The effect was amazing. We got the men and women up to dance, taught them a few belly dance moves and did some collective head-banging. The women dressed up in our hip-scarves and we all had a great time. Afterwards, I chatted to some of them and they were really friendly. 'I didn't see any bikes outside,' I said to one. 'Nah, love, it's winter, innit? We've brought the car.'

But, as I say, cabaret wasn't really my natural habitat; it was the community aspect of dancing that appealed to me, as well as the promotion of belly dance as an art form on a par with other dance forms such as flamenco and Kathak. To that end, I got involved in the JWAAD teacher training programme; I wanted would-be dancers to learn not only how to do the movements but also the rich cultural context which had given rise to this dance form, which had captivated so many women over the centuries.

Then, in 2002, my perfect life unravelled. I was working so hard that I had a major meltdown. There were sweeping redundancies at work – including some very close friends – and my whole department was restructured. Those of us left took on more and more work and I just couldn't cope. My relationship wasn't working but I didn't want to end it because I was so attached to my partner's two children. I was crying all the time, suffering regular panic attacks and dreaded waking up in the morning. I started seeing a counsellor and was signed off work for three months. I was horrified at the prospect and felt a complete failure. But she insisted. As she said in her letter to my GP:

> Yvette has been worn out by all the changes at work and coped by taking on more outside interests to fulfil her needs. However, coping with a relationship, two jobs, a course and a social life has taken its inevitable toll. She needs a complete break so she can de-stress a bit, get back to a good sleep pattern and be more realistic about how many hours there are in the day!

Having that time off made me really reassess my life. I was a director, with a wardrobe full of designer clothes, a Rolodex of VIP contacts, and the benefits of a generous expense account and all the other perks of a high-status job, but I just wasn't enjoying any of it. I knew that I should be grateful to have such a great job, and I loved working with my authors and seeing their books come to fruition, but thanks to the increasingly heavy workload it had lost its appeal. Besides, my job had changed in the restructure; I was given responsibility for 'Special Projects' – a non-role that really was just one step away from redundancy. So, emboldened by my enforced break, I opted to get out, and made a decision that anybody in my situation would do – to move to south-west France and set up a belly dance school.

With hindsight, it was a reckless move, but then I have never been somebody to do things by halves. And I really wasn't thinking clearly; my head was too full of sequins and sparkles to worry about thoroughly researching the project and putting together a viable business plan. I had visions of sharing my passion for belly dance with young and old, and empowering them to enjoy the sensual moves and feel good about themselves. I was spurred on in my fantasy world by my dear friend Yvonne, who lived there and was overjoyed at the prospect of having me as a neighbour.

Of course, it didn't quite turn out as planned. Marmande – self-proclaimed 'Capital of the Tomato' – wasn't the ideal location for a belly dance school. What might have worked in a buzzing, cosmopolitan city like Paris or Toulouse didn't cut it in this sleepy market town, then in the throes of an economic recession. A place where anything foreign was viewed with some suspicion, and there was no great love of Arabs, let alone their culture.

I arrived in Marmande in January 2003. It was extremely cold and wet and the glorious sunshine and outdoor lifestyle that I remembered so fondly from my previous visits were a distant memory. The flat I had bought was uninhabitable, the builders nowhere to be seen, and as Yvonne's mill had flooded, we were both forced to sleep on the floor in a friend's barn.

Instead of running a dance school, I ended up taking a series of unlikely jobs, just to cover the bills. My first was a foray into selling home-cleaning products – not a huge success as I'd only just arrived in France and nobody I knew would host a party at their home and buy enough products to make it worthwhile. Nor was cleaning exactly my forte. My 90-year-old neighbour, Edith, kindly obliged, but she and all her friends then spent the entire afternoon dismissing the cleaning properties of the various liquids and creams and saying how they swore by newspaper and vinegar. When I offered Edith a six-month supply of cleaner for the price of three, she just shrugged and said, 'But why? I may be dead by then.' Not an auspicious start.

Then I got a job working in the wine shop of a local vineyard. It was just for the minimum wage, but I was thankful for anything. Anyway, I fondly imagined that I would spend my time doing *dégustations* or wine-tastings for the many visitors to the region – but they turned out to be few and far

Yvette Cowles

between in the winter months. I did do some but the bulk of my time was spent filling 33-litre *cubits* with wine from a kind of petrol pump. And, as I was the most junior member of staff and not to be trusted with cashing up at the end of the day, it was my job to mop the floor. It was quite a change from the glittering launch parties and hob-nobbing with the likes of Jeffrey Archer, Margaret Thatcher and Martin Amis. But the locals were very friendly, some of them excessively so; they pinched my cheek and referred to me affectionately as *la petite anglaise*. I felt more like a teenager doing work experience than a 40-year-old woman with years of experience at work. I remember two elderly farmers vying for my attention one day. 'You know, I can give you many sheep,' said one. 'Ah yes, but only I can offer you the finest potatoes in Lot-et-Garonne,' said the other.

Even if the dance school never materialised, to my relief I did manage to do some dancing. When I first arrived, I had contemplated getting a job dancing at a local Moroccan restaurant, but my recently acquired French boyfriend (henceforth MFB) was aghast at the idea. 'This is not respectable in Marmande! Do you want to start life here with a bad reputation?' Even Yvonne, whom I had first met on a belly dance course in Sheffield, admitted that it might not be the best way to introduce myself to the locals. To be honest, I wasn't that upset about it as I didn't like restaurant dancing that much – but I could have done with the income.

But Yvonne was determined to get me dancing again and did all she could to get me work. Thanks to her efforts, I started weekly classes in Bordeaux, Marmande and the village of Levignac, where I had to attend a meeting of the local cultural association. In the church hall I was introduced to the good people of Levignac as 'our new belly dance and hip-hop teacher'. That was news to me! I discovered that I would be teaching this to children aged 8–15. Hip-hop was really not my area of expertise, so I had to improvise. I went to classes at my local gym and passed on what I knew to the children, blending it with Arabic, Bollywood and dance moves of my own creation. 'This is very different hip-hop,' said one girl. '*Bien sûr*,' I said, with my best Gallic shrug. 'It's the English version.'

On one occasion, I even had the opportunity to dance at the grand Casino in Biarritz. Once again, it was thanks to Yvonne, who knew a Moroccan woman whose son was a musician. He was putting on a *spectacle* in Biarritz and one of the dancers had damaged her back. Obviously, Yvonne volunteered my services. I was as terrified as I had been the first time Naget thrust a hip-scarf at me; the other dancers were big names in the French Arabic dance scene and I felt totally inadequate. The auditorium was immense, and I'd never danced in public with a full

Arabic band – or in front of a predominantly Arabic audience of around 500 people. The day didn't start too well either; Yvonne and I managed to get locked out of the building and had to scale a wall to get back in. I fell and twisted my ankle. Then there was only a brief rehearsal with the musicians, whose version of the songs was nothing like the CD I'd been given to listen to beforehand. I was told to just get on with it. And so I did. And it turned out to be one of the most exhilarating nights of my life.

The musicians were flown in from Paris especially for the event. They were an eight-strong band, comprising a singer, *nay* (Egyptian flute), violin, *kanoun*, accordion and keyboards, with the *tabla* and *duff* making up the percussion section. I was performing a *magency* or entrance piece, followed by a much-loved Egyptian song called *Lissa Fakir*, written for Om Kalthoum, Egypt's most celebrated singer. The piece is in the repertoire of all the greatest Egyptian dancers – Fifi Abdou included – and I was anxious to do it justice. I shivered nervously in the wings. I felt sick. But at least I looked like a professional dancer; my jewel-encrusted dress was an Egyptian original and Yvonne had excelled herself with my hair and make-up. As I looked out at the dark auditorium, I couldn't see any faces but I could feel their presence. The stage was large, with the imposing columns of an ancient Egyptian temple as backdrop. Then the orchestra started playing the introduction. I used those bars to take a few deep breaths before entering the stage with my veil held aloft, the air beneath it making it float and shimmer behind me. As I did I chided myself for my nerves, 'How many dancers dream of this opportunity? Just think "Fifi", go with the flow and you'll be fine.'

So I did. Adrenaline kicked in and the pain in my ankle vanished. Dancing with a live band forced me to be totally present, focusing on what the musicians were playing at that precise moment. I knew the music so well that I had certain 'benchmarks' to hold on to, but there was no question of trying to remember complicated choreography or to plan what to do next. I just had to feel the music and connect to the emotion. There was an unpredictability that was both dangerous and thrilling.

Lissa Fakir, meaning 'Do you still remember?', is a very beautiful and emotional piece about a failed love affair; it embraces sorrow and regret but also strikes a note of defiance. During the song there was an improvised solo – *taxsim* – played on the violin, one of my favourite instruments. As in jazz or blues, it's an opportunity for the musician to display his virtuosity. In this case, the violinist had only arrived at the theatre about half an hour before the start of the show and we'd had no chance to rehearse together. I felt totally unprepared. I needn't have worried though; his playing was stunning, and as I oozed and undulated to its rise and fall, with the audience singing along and vocalising their appreciation, I felt as though I was channelling a beautiful, feminine tradition that was as old as the Nile. It was a wonderful experience and the memories of that evening will remain with me forever.

Sadly, though, it was also an experience never to be repeated during my time in Marmande. My daily life was much more mundane – and exhausting too. Although I had made my home there, and made lots of friends there too, money – or rather lack of it – was always a problem. I was teaching dance, running classes in business English, working at the vineyard – but still spending every penny on trying to make my flat even habitable. So after a couple of years in France I returned to England, with MFB in tow. As luck would have it, a former colleague was looking for maternity cover at his publishing house in Stroud, and Hazel Kayes, a fellow belly dancer who I knew vaguely through a friend of a friend, agreed to let us rent a room in her house. I was quite relieved as my father wasn't well and I wanted to be closer to home.

Chapter 4

Cancer – Round Two!

I loved my time in Stroud. Not only was Hazel a great dancer and lovely person, but she was also the most fantastic cook. It was glorious to come home to the aroma of yet another gourmet meal. Even MFB had to admit that her food was amazing. And he was most dismissive of English cuisine; other than cooked breakfasts and cream teas, everything was *dégueulasse*. In fact, he was dismissive of English culture in general; nothing could compare with his beloved France. But then, this was a man who refused to listen to Abba because he deemed 'Waterloo' to be an unpardonable slur on the French. As I said, though, MFB adored Hazel – and her food. More importantly, Hazel became a true friend and was to provide me with tremendous support when I really needed it.

Whatever the drawbacks of my time in rural France, I did return to England fitter and in better shape than at any other time in my life. The outdoor lifestyle, regular workouts in the gym, teaching and

performing dance – not to mention lifting and carrying endless crates of wine – had worked wonders for
my figure! I felt good about myself and optimistic
about the future.

Once again I was working back in publishing and
combining it with teaching dance classes and workshops around the country. I had missed publishing;
although working on a vineyard had been great for
the body, it wasn't over-stimulating for the brain. I
was also making the weekly journey to London to
rehearse with Johara, Jo Wise's new dance company,
and see my parents. Life was busy but nowhere near
as stressful as before. Stroud was a beautiful place
and I loved living in the English countryside; life was
certainly easier than in rural France.

But, by this stage, my father's health was deterio-
rating. He had prostate cancer, and suffered a series
of minor strokes. In February 2006, he had a fall,
from which he never really recovered. His time in
hospital reflected the very worst of the NHS, in
marked contrast to my own treatment. The geriat-
ric wing of his local hospital was dirty and uncared-
for and the staff were indifferent and lacking any
kind of compassion. The whole atmosphere was
one of neglect. My father was so desperate to leave
that he managed to get out of the ward unnoticed
and when my mother came to visit nobody knew
where he was. He was found by visitors in the
hospital car park, wandering round in his pyjamas

in the pouring rain, totally disorientated and in great distress.

A month later my father was dead. He died of a brain aneurysm, sitting in his armchair, watching *Deal or No Deal* on TV. It was exactly the way he would have wanted to go, but it was heartbreaking for my mother who found him there, having just made her third phone call to their GP, whom she'd been pleading with to come and visit him because he was in such pain.

When I received the news in Stroud I couldn't believe it. I was in regular contact with my parents and had only spoken to Dad the day before. I was certainly in no fit state to drive up to London on my own so Hazel came with me. I adored my father, who was one of the kindest and most caring men you could hope to meet – 'a true gentlemen', as his friends always described him. I just couldn't deal with his passing so I did what I always did in unbearable situations; I blotted it out and kept myself as busy as possible.

I became quite obsessive about exercising and staying in shape and I was concerned when, a few months later, I noticed a lesion on my nipple and marks around the breast and went to my local GP. 'It's nothing,' he reassured me, 'probably just a scratch and a fungal infection.' He prescribed me some cream, but the lesion didn't go away, so I made an appointment at the Royal Marsden.

Yvette Cowles

I had been signed off by the hospital only a few months before at my annual check-up. It was 2006 – 10 years after my lumpectomy – and I was judged to be low-risk. I had been told that I needn't come back any more, except to have an annual mammogram, or if I had any concerns. It had been quite a relief.

I had my tests and then went for the results to the Breast Diagnostic Unit at the hospital, by now in a state-of-the-art new building. I saw one of my consultant Mr Gui's team. For some reason, I wasn't unduly concerned, so had gone for the appointment on my own. (Note to all cancer patients – never, never do that! You need someone with you, not just for moral support but to fully absorb exactly what is being said in case you can't.) The doctor explained that the cancer had returned and that, given that this was a recurrence, the recommended course of action would be a mastectomy followed by a course of chemotherapy. I couldn't believe what I was hearing. I remember passing out and coming to on a trolley. I was quite dazed, but tried to get up. I needed to get out of there. The consultant looked concerned. 'We can't let you go home on your own. Isn't there someone who could come and collect you?' MFB was driving an HGV somewhere around Europe and my friends were either working or some distance away. I thought of my mother. She was 75 and it would be a tube journey up to the hospital

34

from North London, but I knew she wouldn't mind. So I called her and she came immediately. Meanwhile, the kindly breast care nurse made me a cup of tea. I thought of all those British kitchen sink dramas and how the kettle always went on in times of crisis.

Within a matter of days I was back at the hospital for my operation, with my mother and MFB in tow. I found the ward and settled myself in. MFB was astonished. 'Don't you have your own room?' he asked. 'No, this is the NHS,' I told him, 'and besides, I think I'd prefer to have company. I can always draw the curtains round if I want some privacy.' My boyfriend launched into a tirade about the inadequacies of the English health system in comparison with that of his beloved France. It wasn't particularly helpful given that I wasn't being treated in France. My mother bristled. When he went off in search of a coffee, she warned me, 'Yvette, do tell him to shut up, or I will *hit* him.' As I knew he would be staying with her in North London for the next few days, I was rather alarmed. But I figured that they would have to sort themselves out; I had more pressing concerns to worry about.

The following day my breast was marked up – after all, it would have been rather upsetting to lose the wrong one – and I was put on a trolley ready to go down to the operating theatre. Just I was about to go, there was a phone call for me. 'Yvette, I hope I'm not too late. I'm sending you love and healing light,' said a breathless voice. 'Just imagine you're going on a beautiful journey towards good health and well-being.' I was mystified. Who *was* this? Then suddenly it clicked. It was the lovely Jill Chartell, from the good old Belly Dance-In days, whom I'd barely seen since. It was so incongruous that I burst out laughing and chuckled all the way down to theatre.

I awoke after the op in the recovery room. I looked down and saw that my breast had gone. No padding, nothing but a thin strip of tape over a now completely flat surface. So much for breaking it to me gently! I wasn't upset, though; the cancer had obviously been growing pretty rapidly. By the time I had the surgery my breast looked puckered and diseased; I just wanted to be rid of it. I would have liked reconstruction at the time, but my consultant strongly advocated waiting. The cancer was obviously quite aggressive and the team wanted to be clearer about what they were dealing with before building me a new breast.

The day after surgery I was bombarded with phone calls, cards and visitors. I had an impassioned call from MFB's mother, '*Ma chère* Madeleine, you must absolutely *not* have this operation in England! My son tells me that your hospitals are worse than in Africa! You must come back to France!' I had to break the news to her that it was a little late for that.

Belly Dancing and Beating the Odds

I should explain that MFB and his family insisted on calling me by my middle name, 'Madeleine'. This was because, while Yvette is quite an exotic and unusual name in Britain, it is the French equivalent of 'Doreen', last popular during the Second World War, and so deeply unfashionable as far as MFB was concerned. And, of course, he had his reputation as a suave, sophisticated Frenchman to consider. (Incidentally, the name change didn't go down very well with my mother, whose name actually is Doreen!)

My friends and family rallied round as before. MFB did his best, but he was completely thrown by the whole episode. His life experience did not equip him with the skills to deal with a girlfriend with cancer. Although he had got work and made friends in spite of speaking very little English, he found life here difficult and unsettling. He relied on me to be the strong one who would look after him, not the other way around. His way of coping was to hold my hand in his, look heavenwards and sigh deeply. 'Ah, *mon bon Dieu*, what 'ave we done to deserve *zees*?' I didn't blame him, but it wasn't very helpful, so I was relieved when he had to go back to work and I could go back and recuperate at my mother's house in peace.

Having had breast cancer herself, my mother understood perfectly. I needed to rest and not worry about supporting somebody else through my illness.

She cosseted me and made me endless cups of tea. Besides, there was the question of follow-up treatment to consider. Although, thankfully, my lymph nodes were clear, my consultant was keen for me to have a course of chemotherapy to eradicate any rogue cells that might still be there.

Chemotherapy – my worst fear. I had heard so much about the side-effects: the nausea, the overwhelming fatigue, the hair loss. It was the last thing I needed. And, furthermore, there was the risk to fertility. I was already over 40 and my chances of having children were growing less and less likely. Prior to the operation I was told that I could have some eggs frozen but that it would delay the surgery by a few weeks – something that the consultant was very reluctant to do. However, they did give me regular injections of Zoladex, designed to protect my ovaries. Zoladex: the same drug that was given to my father to keep his prostate cancer in check.

I knew I was lucky that the cancer, although aggressive, had not spread, but nevertheless I felt really low. Although these precautions were taken to protect my ovaries, I was told that the treatment combined with my age made having a baby extremely unlikely. That was a real blow. But at times when I felt really low and too exhausted to see anyone, I once again turned to belly dance; I put on cheerful, uplifting music and just allowed myself to move as much or as little as I wanted.

Belly Dancing and Beating the Odds

I started chemo just before Christmas. The nurses had told me that I could wear a cold cap during treatment to help prevent hair loss. It looked like a padded swimming cap but felt as though my head had been plunged into an ice bucket. Once was enough; from then on I thought I'd take my chances without. My hair started to thin out initially and then to come out in uneven clumps. I'd wake up to find it on the pillow, on my clothes, in my mouth. It was quite depressing, both for me and for my mother, who took it particularly badly. When she had cancer she had a lumpectomy and radiotherapy, but no chemo. I only had to look at the expression on her face to know that I wasn't looking at my best. 'You know, given the choice, I would rather lose my breast than lose my hair,' she said, looking at my bald head sadly. I couldn't quite understand her rationale. Admittedly, in my hair-free state I looked less like the glamorous Lieutenant Ilia from *Star Trek* and more Mr Potato Head, but as I said to her, 'Mum, at least hair grows back.'

Fortunately, my belly dance friends came to the rescue once more. Margaret (the friend who, if you recall, had brought me the inflatable man, first time round) marched me off to a local wigmakers. Belly dancers are used to wearing hairpieces and wigs, so I spent an afternoon trying on different styles. Should I go for a completely new look – long, dark and sultry *à la* Cher? Or perhaps launch myself as a fiery redhead? Or go for full-on Dolly Parton glamour? In the end, I bought several – including one that wasn't too dissimilar to my usual look. In any case, they were all preferable to the ones the NHS had to offer, which were alarmingly shiny and synthetic looking bouffant creations; quite possibly all the rage circa 1970 but certainly not since.

I continued to work part-time for the publishers in Stroud, but the start of my chemotherapy coincided with a takeover by the company's former owner. My colleagues – particularly those who had worked with this man in the past – were distraught and the general atmosphere was one of gloom and despondency. I adopted my usual role of trying to look on the positive side, but it was an uphill struggle. Being in that working environment was not what I needed, and it was a relief to escape to London, spend time with my mother and start dancing again.

One of the first events I went to was the Fantasia Festival in London; it was popular with belly dancers as it offered a wide range of workshops plus an emporium of costumes, scarves, music and anything else that a dancer could desire. I walked into the *souk* (as the bazaar is known) and saw women trying on gorgeous, glittery costumes, dresses with plunging necklines or two-piece outfits with beautifully decorated bras, and knew that I would never be able to wear one again. Suddenly I felt overwhelmed by everything – the chemo, the mastectomy, having cancer for the second time – and I had to get out of there. It was all too much.

And now that I was lacking one, I became aware of breasts being flaunted everywhere – on billboards, on Page 3, in everyday life. There were creams to make them perkier, cleavage-enhancing clothes and bras to lift, separate and boost your boobs by a few cup sizes. And if the natural version wasn't to your taste, there was always silicone. Unless, of course, you were me; I wasn't allowed to have a replacement one for the time being.

But those moments of sorrow and frustration were few and far between. Most of the time I coped, as I always do, by focusing on the positive and trying to push anything unpleasant into the darkest recesses of my mind. I was lacking a breast, but at least the asymmetric look had come back into fashion. And I told myself that I was just following in the tradition of the Amazons, a race of mighty warrior women, who had one breast removed so it wouldn't jeopardise their hunting prowess by preventing them from drawing a bow and arrow.

MFB returned to France. He was coming under pressure from his family to return home and get involved in the family's viticulture business, and he thought that once he'd got himself established, I would follow him. But I didn't. Being ill had made me realise just how much I needed to be in familiar surroundings, with my friends and family. My dreams of creating a family with him had long since evaporated, and our relationship was just not strong enough to survive the physical and emotional fallout from cancer. I had discovered that even the most ardent Francophile eventually reaches her Waterloo.

Chapter 5

Cancer - Round Three!

Before, dancing had played second fiddle to my career in publishing, but now I knew that life was too precious to waste doing something when my heart and soul craved something else. I wanted to dance – and to encourage other women to do the same.

So I decided to leave publishing and focus on dancing, but I realised that I needed to have a back-up if I wasn't able to work. I joined a group designed to help women find 'financial freedom' through different ways of generating 'passive income'. It all made sense at the time, and prompted me to get involved in several different schemes. Unfortunately, as I later discovered to my cost, for one reason or another not one of them would be successful, and those very investments, which were designed to give me more financial security, actually did the very opposite. It took me a while to fully appreciate the old adage 'if it looks too good to be true, it probably is', but it certainly proved to be correct in my case. And as anyone working with cancer patients will tell you, when you're going through, or even emerging from, the emotional fallout of cancer, it's not a time to be making major decisions that will impact on your future. You're not in the right head space for that. Well, I certainly wasn't; post-chemo my brain was definitely pure mashed potato!

I started working for a lifestyle company in Cheltenham, completely unrelated to publishing. Originally, it was designed to be a holistic centre offering different therapies and coaching, and I liked and trusted the people involved. I was going to teach belly dance and co-ordinate the dance programme there. But it wasn't financially viable, and through necessity the company was forced to abandon therapies in favour of teeth whitening, medical cosmetics and makeover photo-shoots. It was neither my area of expertise nor something that particularly interested me. And the constant upheaval and day-to-day challenges of keeping the company afloat were draining and certainly not conducive to a calm and stress-free life. It was absolutely not what I needed, but by then I had already become a director and invested a substantial amount in the company – money that I soon realised I would have been better off keeping in the bank for a rainy day. I felt trapped.

My love life was equally problematic. It was hard to meet men anyway given the circles I moved in, and online dating seemed fraught with danger. How should I go about meeting someone? At what point should I mention that I only had one breast? How would the person respond? Would they run away screaming? In fact I got a variety of responses: 'Ouch, that must have hurt!' and 'You're OK, I'm more of a bum man really!' being just a couple of them. And one man did seem to have what I considered to be an unnatural fixation with the surgical procedure behind my mastectomy. It was most off-putting. And so, after a few efforts, I decided that I was better off on my own.

I continued to go to the Marsden for my annual mammogram. Like most women, I hated them. At least, as I consoled myself, they were less uncomfortable now as I only had one breast to squidge and squeeze into position. But then, in 2010, following the mammogram I was surprised to receive a call from the consultant. She said because the mammogram had revealed a 'benign change in tissue', they would arrange for me to have an ultrasound scan. I was suffering from a bad cold at the time and found it hard to take in. 'Does that mean cancer?' I asked. I heard a pause on the end of the phone. 'Well, the appearances are not consistent with cancer, but we need to be sure.'

A few days later I was back at the Marsden, having an ultrasound. This time I'd learned my lesson; I took my mother with me. During the course of the procedure, the friendly radiographer's face suddenly changed; she looked serious and muttered, 'Ah, this is more sinister than I thought.' She offered me a biopsy and I had it right away. By then, tears were streaming down my face. I clutched my mother's hand and saw that she was crying too. Surely, I thought, not again? But the radiographer was non-committal. It would be up to my consultant to give me the results.

I returned to the Royal Marsden the following day to see Mr Gui, my lovely caring consultant, with a penchant for natty ties. He looked genuinely sad to see me again, and told me that the cancer had come back and that I should follow the same procedure as before – that is, a mastectomy and chemotherapy. My first thought: at least I know what to expect. And my second: at least now I'll be symmetrical.

The following Monday I went to the pre-assessment clinic – blood test, MRSA swab, ECG, blood test, anesthetist check up, and finally, a visit to the medical photographer. I was pointed in the direction of a corridor in the wing of the hospital that was at the time under renovation. I picked my way through the plastic sheeting and past the workmen and found myself in a dark and dingy little room. I had to remove my top and bra. Waiting for me was a man in a white coat and glasses with a camera. He was a medical photographer, whose job was to photograph me from six different angles, including my back, just in case I had back flap reconstruction at some point.

Funnily enough, only the week before, one of my belly dance buddies and I had been for a makeover photo-shoot at a studio in Cheltenham. We'd taken a selection of costumes, been given the five-star treatment, with champagne and a session with our very own stylist and photographer. The results were amazing; I looked like one of those Egyptian dancers whom I'd watched so avidly on screen, and I could hardly believe that, with the help of good lighting and some judicious touching up, I had been trans-formed into such a glamorous creature. But not this time; it was clear that the Royal Marsden Hospital favoured a strictly no-frills approach.

The following day I went to the hospital for my operation. I had to be there by 7.30am, and as it was snowing heavily, I told my mother not to come. I got a mini-cab, and ironically, the driver was a woman who'd taken me on several previous occasions to Wood Lane, when my authors were being inter-viewed on *BBC Breakfast*. She started on the same route this time round and I had to put her right. This time my destination was a hospital rather than a TV studio. In fact, the days of PR and author tours seemed a lifetime away.

I arrived and was left in a cubicle. I was issued with delightful surgical stockings, and an even more fetching back-opening gown. I wasn't sure how long I'd be there, but when a kindly nurse wheeled in an ancient TV, especially for me, I had an inkling that I would be in for a fairly long wait. As I sat there, semi-comatose, it occurred to me that, with NHS cuts in place, perhaps now daytime TV was being used to anaesthetise patients. If so, it was definitely working.

Around 2.30pm, my consultant Mr Gui and his registrar, Sasha, came round. I remember thinking that he had surpassed himself with his choice of tie that day. It was bright, even by my standards. My breast was marked up – though this time they could hardly get the wrong one – and I was wheeled down to theatre. Funnily enough, I didn't feel any attachment to my remaining breast.

But being breast-less – or about to be – and the removal of lymph nodes in the other armpit, did mean that I no longer had a 'good' arm. Because of the risk of lymphoedema, the blood pressure pad had to be put around my calf, and when it contracted it was extremely painful. I also had to have the canula put in my foot rather than my hand. Again, it was not a pleasant experience. But very soon I drifted off and didn't feel a thing.

I came round at about 4.30pm. I was wide-awake and felt no discomfort, though I felt a bit cheated that I wasn't offered morphine as my blood pressure was low. I'd enjoyed that warm drowsy feeling the last time round. My mother had braved the snow to come and visit and I thought I'd use the opportunity to unpack my bags and rearrange the seating a bit, much to the nurse's horror. She forced me back to bed and brought us both a cup of tea. Tea, the ultimate panacea! I instantly felt better.

The ward was small and friendly but hardly conducive to a good night's sleep, thanks to the combination of the sauna-like temperature, my snoring fellow patients, clanking machines and the regular visits of nurses to check your blood pressure and issue painkillers.

The next day was one of frenzied cleaning activity in the ward. Being the first of the month, it was time to flip the mattresses, so that at least caused a bit of diversion. Then there was the older woman in the bed directly opposite, who was very friendly but insisted on remaining naked beneath her hospital gown. She kept bending down and flashing her nether regions to anyone unfortunate enough to be looking in her direction, which was often me as she was directly in my line of vision. It was particularly disconcerting at mealtimes. I was grateful for my selection of 'lounge wear' (as my mother quaintly described it), which I'd customised with sequins. I'd stuffed the gown into my locker; there was no way that *I* would be mooning at anyone.

Over the next few days I had a succession of visitors again – many of them my dance friends – whom I took to the hospital café. The nurses were rather bemused by the constant to-ing and fro-ing, and one warned me that if I continued at this rate, the hospital would have to issue me with my very own pager. But my visitors appreciated it. Funnily enough, they said that they hadn't seen me look so good in ages, and other patients I met on my regular cappuccino trips asked me whom I had come to visit, which just goes to show the power of regular meals and complete bed rest.

I had been given some physiotherapy exercises to do, which I embraced wholeheartedly. Being a breast-free belly dancer was one thing, but one who couldn't use her arms was quite another. I was anxious to get my full range of movement back as quickly as possible. While some of my fellow patients couldn't be bothered, I did the exercises 20, 30, 40 times a day, drawing the curtains around my cubicle to avoid being scolded. I soon got bored of the hospital versions so I invented my own, which obviously had a belly-dance twist. I even encouraged my fellow patients to join me. However, Sasha, the registrar, soon got wise to this and she and one of the nurses of the ward took to surprising me and making us stop.

When I was finally sent home, I felt well, but that night I had what my mother would call 'a funny turn'. I had a curious pain in my chest and felt very sick. As I tried to get to the bathroom I fainted and hit my head on the bedroom door. I reluctantly woke up my mother and she changed my dressing as the wound was really beginning to swell. I called the hospital and they told me to come in first thing in the morning.

At the hospital I saw Sasha. As I came into the room she said to the nurse with her, 'This is the theatrical one I was telling you about', and asked me sternly if I had been 'flinging, flapping or flailing my arms' when I fainted. She looked very dubious when I protested that I had just been in bed, writing my diary. But Mr Gui confirmed that the wound just hadn't drained off properly. I was triumphant; it had nothing whatsoever to do with over-exercising!

The next step was another course in chemotherapy, this time an accelerated one. I was apprehensive, but at least this time I knew what to expect. I asked a friend to give me a number one cut so that the inevitable hair loss would be less traumatic, and dusted off the wigs from last time round.

Then, just a few days before I started, I received a phone call. I had invested a substantial amount of my savings in a property scheme but the capital was due to be returned to me in just a few weeks. The property developer told me that he didn't have the money to repay me, and couldn't tell me when he would get the funds either. I was devastated. Not this on top of everything else. I couldn't tell my mother or brother; I was too ashamed of my stupidity and didn't want to cause them unnecessary stress. I felt totally alone. Alone, that is, until I found out that I was far from being this man's only victim. It emerged that there were a number of us – mainly women – who'd lost large sums of money investing in his scheme. And at least we were able to support each other during the upsetting times ahead.

But for the time being I pushed those problems to the back of my mind. I needed to keep what energy and mental strength I had for my treatment. Not only that, but Johara Dance Company was busy rehearsing for a string of theatre shows, and I was determined to be well enough to perform. My mother was anxious about the stress of it all, but I needed a goal to get me through eight weeks of chemotherapy.

And it did. At times it was hard, though. On one occasion, we had a photographer lined up to take publicity shots of us to use for the show. That morning I looked at myself in the mirror. I had folliculitis, so my bald head was covered in itchy red spots, I had no eyebrows or eyelashes, my eyes were bloodshot, I looked pale and drawn, and my teeth were a rather unattractive brown colour because of the mouth wash I had to use to ward off ulcers. I couldn't face *that* look being recorded for posterity, so I made my excuses and stayed at home.

But that was the only time. Other than that, I dutifully turned up at every rehearsal, even if I didn't have the energy to do much dancing. It was a kind of therapy for me. I loved moving my body in such a familiar way, even if my shimmies were a little less vigorous than usual and my upper body movements a little more cautious. I was involved in a number of group dances as well as a solo. I was anxious that my memory would let me down and that consequently I'd let down my 15 fellow dancers, but they gave me lots of support and understanding. They all knew how much the show meant to me.

I was worried about them seeing my scars too. We had a number of quick costume changes and it just wasn't possible to preserve your modesty. We had to fling our clothes off and put new ones on in a matter of minutes. In contrast to all the bouncing breasts around me, I was completely flat-chested, with a sheer drop from collarbone to navel and a couple of scars where my breasts had once been. Initially, I felt desperately self-conscious. But nobody batted an eyelid, and that total acceptance was just what I needed.

In fact being 'breast-free' had its advantages. I was now perfectly symmetrical, and no longer had to stress about their shape or size. Mine would never go southwards and end up around my knees. And anyway, with the help of prostheses or 'comfies' stuffed down my bra I could go for any look I liked, from gamine Audrey Hepburn to pneumatic Jayne Mansfield. What's more, men now looked into my eyes when they spoke to me, and it certainly put my cellulite into perspective.

But I did – and still do – miss my breasts. Even now, I have a recurring dream in which my breasts are giant pink helium balloons that keep on floating away from me. I devise more and more elaborate ways of stopping them – from multiple bras and ropes and pulleys to the Thames Barrier itself – but they still slip from my grip and float away from me.

But it turned out breasts – or rather the lack of them – was the least of my worries. Tests revealed that the cancer had spread to the lymph nodes and bone. I was devastated. This particular bombshell was thrown into a conversation with a doctor while I was having chemo. She obviously thought I already knew, but I didn't. In fact, the last set of scans appeared to show that the disease had been contained. In that moment everything changed. Suddenly my conversations with the medical team revolved around ways of 'stabilising' the disease, rather than 'curing' it. I was told that cancer was something I would have to live with, rather like diabetes. 'Don't worry,' said the consultant, 'we'll keep an eye on you so that when it flares up again we can act quickly.' That wasn't exactly reassuring – what did they mean, '*When* it flares up again'? Whatever happened to *if*?

From now on I would be a regular at the Royal Marsden, with monthly infusions to protect my bones, blood tests, plus scans every few months. I was certainly getting my money's worth from the NHS. I realised that this time round I wouldn't experience that sense of being cast adrift and left to cope on my own, as cancer patients often feel when the treatment ends. I'd felt that myself after Cancers One and Two. It wasn't true, of course, as the medical team was always there to turn to if there was a problem, but it's unsettling to lose the regular appointments that became part of the fabric of your life.

My mother generally came to appointments with me; she considered herself my lucky charm. I was very grateful for her support. We were a strange double act whom Professor Smith and his oncology team seemed to find very entertaining. Whereas I loathed medical procedures, particularly anything involving needles, she found them fascinating. I just put it down to all her years of sewing. On one occasion I found her crouching under the bed trying to get a better view of the nurse putting a canula in my foot. (A canula is a small tube used to give injections or to take blood.) She was in her element at the hospital, and rated the different departments by the quality – and quantity – of the cups of tea they provided.

Initially, given her age, hospital staff assumed that she was the patient, which caused her immense frustration. Furthermore, she never appreciated the tendency to call her by her first name, Doreen. 'It's *Mrs Cowles*, to you!' she regularly protested. 'Honestly, why are people so *matey*, nowadays?'

Like my belly dance buddies, my mother has been the constant throughout my treatment. In spite of our very different attitude to life, she is my 'rock' and the person I love most in the world. Over the years, I've provided her with more than her fair share of worries, both through my medical mishaps and, as far as she is concerned, my bizarre behaviour and incomprehensible lifestyle choices – but she has still always been there for me.

My mother has the memory of an elephant, whereas mine rivals that of a goldfish with amnesia. Mum's memory can be a bit tedious at times, since she can remember every one of my misdemeanours since birth, but it does also have its upside. Nothing gets past her. And, as I've mentioned, that's a big asset for any cancer patient.

One time I went to the Royal Marsden to see the consultant and, as usual, my mother insisted on coming with me. At the end of the consultation, at which we'd had an amiable chat about medication, anaemia, joint pain and summer holidays, the registrar asked my mother if she had any questions. 'Yes,' she said, 'when are you going to give us the results of Yvette's x-ray?' The registrar and I both looked blank. 'You know, the x-ray you did to see if the spot on her lung was anything to worry about!' Mum persisted. Now, that's a fairly major concern, as the lungs are often the next stop for breast cancer after the bones. I had genuinely forgotten ever having the x-ray done, let alone worried about the results, and even though it was one of many procedures I was having at the time, my x-ray amnesia was still rather alarming. However, on the plus side, it had saved me a number of sleepless nights, and allowed me to fill my head with new dances, costumes and fun activities for my students. Maybe being a goldfish has its good points, I thought. I can just blank things out, and leave my mother to be my memory and do the worrying for me, as she's going to do that anyway! (Incidentally, when the registrar checked, the lung was fine.)

One of the most bizarre incidents during all my years of treatment involved my mother – and my foot. Because the cancer is in my lymph nodes and a couple of bones, I have to have regular bone scans. On this one occasion I had to have a CT scan at the Royal Marsden and a bone scan at the Royal Brompton. But as the hospitals are next to each other it all seemed pretty straightforward.

The staff left the canula in my foot to save a new one being put in. But it did mean that I couldn't get my boot back on – and only half a sock. No worries – the hospital was next door. The nurse tried to get me a porter but none was available. 'Really, it's fine,' I said, 'I can make my own way.' The nurse looked rather dubious, but as the waiting room was heaving, I think she was actually quite relieved. And, then again, being a true Brit, I wanted to cause the minimum of fuss.

So I started hopping along the corridor, boot in one hand, mother on my other arm. It did suddenly occur to me that it was going to take longer than I had anticipated. Suddenly a nurse came rushing out of a doorway. 'What *are* you doing?' she demanded. 'I'm hopping to my next appointment', I said, and even as I said it I knew that I was bound to be in breach of Health and Safety regulations. Sure enough, the nurse insisted that I wait for a porter. One turned up, pretty quickly, as it happened – a big burly bloke with a young work experience guy in tow armed with a clipboard.

The trouble was that no one seemed to know where the Department of Nuclear Medicine was at the Royal Brompton. It wasn't next door at all but on another site entirely – at least three blocks away. Now the porter had a dilemma. He wasn't meant to leave the premises but he couldn't just tip me out of the chair. So he decided that the best course of action was to take me to the hospital but get there and back as quickly as possible. So we set off at break-neck speed, the work experience lad in hot pursuit and my mother bringing up the rear.

We careered through the streets of South Kensington, scattering startled pedestrians. I looked round for my mother but couldn't see past the porter. 'Where's my mother?' I asked him anxiously. 'Oh, she's all right,' he said. 'Keep up, keep up!' he shouted, looking over his shoulder at her.

The porter and I arrived at the Brompton, to be greeted by a woman in a pink silk sash. 'Blimey,' I thought, in my slightly dazed state, 'it's Miss Royal Brompton!' It turned out that she was a volunteer. The porter deposited me with some relief, and rocketed off, leaving me hopping on one foot and looking around for another wheelchair.

My mother finally arrived, puffing and wheezing. (She was 81 after all, and hadn't run since her school-days, as far as I'm aware.) Miss Royal Brompton called anxiously for a wheelchair, which miraculously appeared from nowhere. 'No, no,' said Mum in exasperation, pointing to the canula in my foot. '*I'm* not the patient, my daughter is.'

The next problem was how to get me to the Department of Nuclear Medicine. Miss Royal Brompton looked anxious. 'I would push you myself, but it's Health and Safety ...' 'Don't worry' said my mother, 'I'll do it.' I was a little dubious – I knew that my mother's trolley-wheeling skills were even worse than mine. And I was right. We set off and she promptly wheeled me into the lift door. At which point Miss Royal Brompton decided that my mother posed an even greater Health and Safety risk and took the wheelchair herself. 'Good ploy!' I whispered to my mother. 'Humph!' was all she said.

Each time I've been recovering from cancer I've been amazed by the response from other people. Compared with my mother, whose close friends crossed the street rather than face the embarrassment of saying the wrong thing, I've been extremely

Yvette Cowles

lucky. As I've said before, my belly dancing buddies in particular always offered just the right practical and emotional support, and, most importantly, kept me laughing.

Even so, I have still encountered people who ask how I think I've brought the cancer on myself. Worse still, I've heard it attributed to 'karma' or 'God's punishment'. It's human nature to try and find an answer to life's problems and seek an explanation for disease and illness. And cancer is such an emotive word; it's easy for people to project their fears and anxieties about it onto you. But it certainly isn't helpful to make someone who is going through something as traumatic as cancer, feel that they have brought the illness on themselves.

I do believe that we have a part to play in our own wellbeing, through our lifestyle, diet, patterns of behaviour, ways we handle stress and the environment we live in. But it's not the whole picture. We simply can't control everything that happens to us, and to pretend that we can, sets us up for failure and makes us feel guilty and inadequate. And when you're undergoing cancer treatment, that's the last thing you need.

Following Cancer No. 3, I became a bit of a self-help junkie. I started my day by writing my 'morning pages' as suggested in *The Artist's Way* and jotting in my gratitude journal, did a quick meditation, recited affirmations in front of the mirror while brushing my teeth, practised Laughter Yoga in the shower and then settled down to some yoga stretches. By 10am I was completely exhausted and in need of a lie-down. A well-meaning friend and raw food expert had come to stay while I was away, and I returned to find everything in my cupboard labelled with post-its, each with either a smiley or sad face drawn on them and a message. 'Very acidic. Not good for cancer (sad face)' or 'Excellent for achieving pH balance (smiley face)'. The sad faces outnumbered the happy ones by four to one and every time I reached into the cupboard I found another one. It was yet another thing to worry about, and at the time, I didn't have the energy for it. In the end, I realised that instead of trying so hard, I had to do what felt right for *me* at the time. And funnily enough, that was putting on some music and dancing my heart out.

When it comes to dealing with the medical profession, I believe that it's good to maintain some degree of control. From the moment that you hear those dreaded words 'I'm sorry, but we've found something', it's very easy to feel that your body is no longer yours. Suddenly, there are an army of other people who lay claim to it. Surgeons, oncologists, radiographers, nurses – everyone's there to grope, prod, examine, sigh, tut. While your medical condition is getting a huge amount of attention, as a person you feel you're all but disappearing.

You want to shout out, 'I'm more than just my cancer, you know!' From the first time I was diagnosed, I found that the only way to avoid disappearing altogether was to go on the offensive. If this army of people wanted to make my body a battlefield, I was going to be the squadron leader, making sure that they all carried out their roles effectively – albeit a squadron leader in sequins. Naturally.

Chapter 6

Sequins on My Balcony

Over the years, experience has taught me that hospitals have much to offer for those who enjoy the absurd. From those appalling gowns that remove every last vestige of dignity to procedures that appear to make no sense whatsoever, it's often pure comedy gold.

While in hospital and receiving treatment I'd regaled my friends with emails and texts about all the funny, ridiculous and bizarre things that were going on. Several of them, including my good friend and dance teacher, Jo Wise, asked me why I didn't write them down, share them as a talk, or make them into a show. And so the germ of an idea was born.

A friend of mine suggested getting in touch with a life coach, Paul Fuggle, to help me get the project underway. He was exactly what I needed. In contrast to some of the more 'left field' therapies I'd tried, Paul took a practical and systematic approach. He asked the right questions and, by checking in with him at regular intervals, I took at least one small step each day to forward the project. As he predicted, once I got going, it soon gained its own momentum, and the right people came into my life to help me.

I started by giving talks to groups at holistic centres, Women's Institutes and Townswomen's Guilds. I hadn't discussed a lot of what I'd written with anybody before, even my close friends, so I felt very anxious and vulnerable. Not least because the women present were generally over 70 years old and extremely forthright. 'Don't worry, we'll tell you if you're rubbish!' one told me cheerfully.

One of the most memorable occasions was when an elderly lady, June, got up to dance with me at the end of one of my talks. She put a scarf round her hips and really seemed to enjoy herself. Afterwards, the organiser told me that she was 'riddled with cancer' and had only just come back to the club, having been beaten up and raped in her own home. I found her story so distressing that I couldn't get it out of my head; it really made me realise how trivial my own concerns were. If a woman in her eighties could cope with something as appalling as that, then I had no excuse for allowing my anxieties to stand in my way.

Then, through Gosia Gorna, one of the brilliant therapists at The Haven in London, I met a wonderful director and theatre-maker, Peta Lily, herself a breast cancer survivor. Not only did Peta have vast experience working with artists to turn their personal story into theatre or the spoken word, but she had also created her own one-woman show about breast cancer. She agreed to help me create mine. I called it *Sequins on My Balcony: Breasts, Belly Dancing and Beating the Odds*, and hoped it would entertain, inspire and give hope to others going through breast cancer, as well as their friends and families.

The title came from a French expression for a woman with a very big bust – *Il y a du monde au balcon*, that is to say, 'she has a crowded balcony'. Obviously, my balcony was dismantled some time ago courtesy of the Cancer Demolition Company, but it's still there in my head – and covered in sequins.

It was quite a daunting prospect as my performance experience was largely limited to dance. But I was determined to make a go of it and developed new skills by training in clowning, drama and even stand-up comedy. I don't think that Peta was prepared for what she was letting herself in for – my total lack of experience being the biggest obstacle – but she recognised my complete commitment to the project and never gave up on me. Not everyone shared her confidence. Ever the pessimist, and being the most risk-adverse person I know, my mother asked me, 'Why would anybody want to come and see *that*, dear?' But I was confident that they would, and hoped that my experiences might strike a chord in other women.

But then, I always relish a new challenge. I love to develop new skills and broaden my horizons, and I firmly believe that we never stop learning. Laughter yoga, clowning, African dance, not to mention other belly dancers' classes and workshops – all have enriched my life as well as influencing my dancing and teaching. I will always love authentic Egyptian belly dance, but inspired by some of the fantastic fusion dancers coming through on the international scene, I started incorporating other influences, from Bollywood to the Charleston and even vaudeville, into my dancing, creating a more theatrical and individual style. And why not? I think it's essential to keep our minds open because the most unexpected things can come in useful, inspire creativity and take us in new and interesting directions. My mantra is 'Think "Fifi", go with the flow and you'll be fine'. Following your passions is key to a happy and fulfilling life, as far as I'm concerned. And this message is the crux of my show.

My first show would probably never have happened had it not been for my good friend and doyenne of theatre PR, Anne Mayer. She kept asking me if I had a confirmed date for a scratch performance (an early run through of a performance to test the material and technicalities), and I said that I wasn't quite ready. So she took matters into her own hands, contacted Cecilia Darker, director of the

Rosemary Branch Theatre in Islington, and got me a date about two months hence.

Up to that point the show had been something I thought about doing sometime in the future, when I felt totally prepared. This was never going to happen. As usual, people rallied round to help me. Jo's husband, John Gosler, an amazing artist and graphic designer, helped me with the design and production of flyers and publicity material. We were in Arras for the wedding of one of the dance company members. It took place in the idyllic setting of a local château, and we took advantage of the wonderful façade and its impressive balcony to set up pictures of me with an inflatable man – Dick Rogers Mark 2 – much to the bemusement of the other guests.

Valérie Romanin, another dancer friend, generously let Peta and me rehearse in her mirrored studio at home, thus saving on studio costs. And Cecilia gave us days of free rehearsal time in the theatre itself. Tim, a friend of a friend, who had been helping decorate my flat, offered to handle the sound and lighting for me on the night. 'Have you ever done it before?' I asked. 'No, but I've DJ'd a fair bit and I'm a fast learner,' he replied. I was a bit dubious, but I needn't have worried. He was brilliant, coping admirably with the 27 sound cues and various lighting states, the logistics of loading, unloading and setting up all the props, and, as importantly, my extremely frayed nerves!

The multi-talented Vashti once again was there for me, this time offering her services as voiceover. Helen, a friend from Stroud, not only helped me to publicise the event but also agreed to be my on-stage prompt. I was worried that all the chemotherapy I'd had would cause my memory to evaporate when I most needed it. One of its most prevalent side-effects is 'mashed potato brain', and that, combined with the fact that it often brings on early menopause, is a pretty deadly combination.

The first show took place on 11 November 2012, a date forever etched on my brain. I don't think I have ever felt more petrified about anything – well, anything not cancer-related, that is. I was terrified of letting myself down – not to mention all the friends, family and fellow dancers who were coming to support me. I had been rather disappointed that my mother refused to come – apart from her fear that it might be an 'unmitigated disaster', she also was concerned about being made into 'some kind of minor celebrity' – but now I was quite relieved. Worrying about her reaction would have added to my nerves.

As I sat waiting for the audience to take their seats, I tried to remember everything that Peta had taught me: the vocal exercises, visualisation methods, relaxation techniques. My mind went totally blank. What if that happened on stage? I just had to trust that, however unprepared I felt, I would pull it off. After all, I had always been somebody renowned for 'winging it'. Whatever I prepared to do, whether workshops or dances, they never went exactly as I'd planned on the day. Once I was in the moment, there were always surprises, but generally good ones; in fact I found that brilliant and inspirational moments often happened that way. I had to trust that this show would be no different, and not dwell on the fact that there was a lot more at stake than usual!

I made my way to the door of the auditorium. I peeped in and saw that it was packed. I was going to make my way through the audience to the strains of 'Boobs', a comedic number by a fifties singer, Ruth Wallis. Tim looked at me enquiringly to see if I was ready. I took a deep breath and nodded. We were on!

The show itself remains a blur, but I do remember that the moment I got on stage I relaxed. Of course things certainly didn't go exactly according to plan: I forgot lines, I dropped props, my breast balloons exploded unexpectedly, and, thanks to a slow puncture, my inflatable man, Dick Rogers Mark Two, became quite deflated. But it didn't matter. In fact, the audience seemed to enjoy those moments best of all. Helen and I made an entertaining double-act, as she rose valiantly to the challenge of keeping me on track.

Afterwards, there was a Q&A session, at which I got some fantastic feedback. 'Moving, fabulously funny and life-affirming', 'more uplifting than a

Wonderbra!' they said. Most touchingly, one of my
parents' closest friends told me that my father would
have loved it. I was euphoric. Not only had I held an
audience's attention on my own for nearly an hour,
but I had loved doing it! For the first time, I felt
completely at home on stage. As I stood and took a
final bow to a standing ovation, it suddenly occurred
to me, 'Maybe *this* is my purpose, perhaps *this* is
what I'm meant to do.'

Buoyed up by that first performance, I scheduled
in more around the country, helped by the local
dance teacher in the area. I decided to support a
local cancer charity with each performance, and also
to use the tour overall to raise awareness and funds
for Just Because, a registered charity aiming to raise
awareness of breast cancer in Egypt, and promote
early detection, treatment and after-care for women
there.

The charity was set up when a group of dancers
got together to raise funds to pay for breast cancer
treatment for their dance friend and mentor, Sara
Farouk, who lives in Cairo. Sara is well known to
everyone in the belly dance community, and dancers
all over the country rose to the challenge, raising far
more money than the initial cost of her treatment.
Consequently, the decision was taken to set up a
charity to continue to raise funds and make a difference to the lives of all women in Egypt. Egypt –
home of belly dance and destination of choice for

dancers from all over the world. Given my passion for belly dance and desire to help other women who didn't have the good fortune to enjoy the level of diagnosis and treatment I had, what better cause to support with my show?

Chapter 7

Mobility Issues

I loved performing the show and loved the fact that it seemed to resonate with so many other women. Then, in summer 2013, I started to experience increasingly bad joint inflammation and pain. I was first aware of it when I came off stage at the Parabola Theatre in Cheltenham. My hip was excruciatingly painful and within seconds I was transformed into a hobbling 90-year-old, in spite of the fact that I hadn't yet turned 50.

Throughout the summer my condition worsened. I went to the JWAAD annual residential summer school, where I regularly teach, and spent most of the time in bed. Even a hug or a handshake hurt like hell. I couldn't sleep at night because my body ached all over, and I was completely exhausted during the day. I avoided socialising too much because I could see the other women's concern written on their faces. Those who knew I had cancer were particularly alarmed and, I heard later, a couple had even gone to the organiser in floods of tears. (I'm very glad I didn't know that at the time!) Over the coming weeks simple tasks that required lifting or any kind of grip became virtually impossible, and when I walked anywhere my progress was so slow and painful that I had difficulty keeping up with people twice my age with their sticks and Zimmer frames.

I had started teaching a weekly Dance Yourself Happy class at Cancerkin, an excellent breast cancer charity based at the Royal Free Hospital, Hampstead, which offers a wide range of services to enable those living with and beyond breast cancer to feel better about themselves. It was a lovely group of women. Each week we danced, sang to Bob Marley, practised Laughter Yoga and even played a spot of air guitar. Everyone threw themselves into the class with great gusto and it was as much a tonic for me as anybody else. But even this was beginning to be a struggle. I used the fact that it was the summer holidays as an excuse to take a few weeks off, hoping that I would feel better after a break.

But by the beginning of September I could barely walk. I had lost a lot of weight too. The consultants at the Royal Marsden were mystified, and I had numerous tests and scans to see if the cancer had spread further, but they revealed nothing. I felt as though my body was shutting down and was terrified. My GP referred me to a CBT (Cognitive Behavioural Therapy) counsellor, who encouraged me to 'accept my current reality'. But I couldn't. I had been through three rounds of cancer and survived (relatively) intact, and my dancing had sustained me throughout. The thought of not being able to dance any more was unthinkable.

I was particularly anxious about a show I had in Leeds in early September. How would I manage to perform a one-hour solo show that combined belly dance with clowning and physical theatre when I couldn't even walk? My lighting and sound guy, Tim, whom I had also enlisted to help with the logistics of getting both me and the props to the various venues around the country, suggested a modified version where I did most of it sitting down. We tried it out in rehearsal; I struggled to sit down and then found it virtually impossible to get out of the chair again. I couldn't raise my arms above my head either. Things weren't looking good.

My mother was aghast that I was even contemplating going. 'For someone who's supposed to be intelligent, you can be really stupid, Yvette.' I know she was trying to protect me but she didn't understand that I *had* to do the show. Firstly, I knew that Loveday, the dancer who was hosting the Leeds gig, had put in a great deal of time and trouble and had even been rehearsing a dance with some of the cancer patients from the local Haven centre to perform at the show. I couldn't bear to let them down. And secondly, I needed to do it for *myself*, to prove that I was still capable of doing it. The show that had started as a labour of love was now my *raison d'être*.

Once again one of my belly dancing buddies came to the rescue. Kay Taylor, a very long-standing friend and fellow teacher who had hosted one of my first shows in Newcastle, invited me to stay at her mother's in Ponden, Yorkshire, to lessen the journey and make the trip easier. She also offered to be my prompt and help out in any other way, should I need it. Nobody inspires more confidence than Kay; she takes everything in her stride, and her relaxed attitude that weekend was immensely reassuring – 'Ee, don't worry, Yvette – it'll all be fine!'

The journey up was slow and painful. Sitting down for long periods of time just made me stiffen up completely. At one stop at a motorway service station I hobbled up the steps to the entrance. A double-amputee on crutches held the door open for me. 'Are you sure you want to go through with this?' asked Tim. 'Of course. Even if I have to be wheeled onto the stage,' I replied.

Kay's mother, Brenda, was the perfect host. She runs a B&B in the idyllic surroundings of the Yorkshire moors, and her cooking is second to none. Her other guests at the time were on a hiking holiday, and we all shared a relaxing evening together. By the end of the meal, though, I could tell I had stiffened up. I didn't think that hobbling away from the dinner table would inspire confidence in me as a performer, so I waited until everyone else had gone to bed before I shuffled off to mine.

The Leeds show the following day went better than I could have possibly hoped for. I took the rehearsal quite gently but during the actual show my body relaxed, the pain and stiffness evaporated and I managed the veil twirling, and even the back bend and 30-second spin in the final number. It was then that I fully appreciated the power of adrenaline – it's not called 'Dr Theatre' for nothing. And the heavy-duty painkillers definitely helped too. Afterwards, there was a Q&A, which I only found out about in the afternoon. Mindful of previous ones where there had been awkward silences, I just kept on talking. I have no idea what I said, but people seemed to be enjoying it.

I was really touched by one woman's comment that it was the first time she had laughed since she was diagnosed with cancer. And one enthusiastic audience member even told me that her only criticism was that the show was too short and she would have liked to have sat through it all over again! For me, though, just once that evening was quite enough.

I returned to London buoyed up by the success of the show. Nobody in the audience appeared to have noticed my physical limitations and I felt proud that I'd been able to put in a good performance regardless. Unfortunately, I paid for it over the next few days, when the adrenaline had well and truly worn off.

Belly Dancing and Beating the Odds

My condition continued to deteriorate until a blood test at my GP's surgery led to the diagnosis of rheumatoid arthritis. I was referred to a rheumatologist, Professor Callan, at the Chelsea and Westminster Hospital. She examined my swollen joints and confirmed that I was suffering from extremely active rheumatoid arthritis (RA) – one of the markers was at 214, whereas a 'normal' reading was less than 10. She gave me a steroid injection for immediate relief and started me on methotrexate, the standard treatment for RA, right away. I could have hugged her; I was so grateful that something was finally being done.

According to Professor Callan, there was no connection with the cancer, and it was more likely due to hereditary factors. (It was true that my puffy knees and ankles looked just like those of my maternal grandmother, who had suffered from RA for nearly 40 years.) My mother was desperately upset; she had seen how much her mother had suffered over the years, and now her daughter had been diagnosed with the same condition. My grandmother had been stoical to the end, but as my mother kept reminding me (not very helpfully, given the circumstances), when the pain had become too much to bear, she had admitted that 'while RA doesn't kill you, it just makes you wish you were dead.'

She was also dismayed that I had another medical condition to contend with. 'Cancer, and now *this*. It's

77

just not fair, Yvette.' But then life isn't. Have you ever seen that 1960s film *Jason and the Argonauts*? Jason is set endless tasks, seemingly at the whim of the gods. Every time he's conquered one foe another crops up, even more deadly and ferocious. Then the gods get bored and decide to leave him in peace – until the next time, anyway. At times I did feel a bit like Jason, dealing as best I could with the crisis at hand, and wondering what was coming next.

And yet the diagnosis was quite a relief. Of course, it was a blow to be diagnosed with yet another incurable disease, but it wasn't life threatening and at least I now knew why my body had been behaving so strangely. And I had the utmost confidence in Professor Callan. At times, when I had been sitting alone in my flat, I had struggled not to imagine the worst. For me, as with so many people with cancer and other serious medical conditions, financial worries had been a primary source of concern. I knew that I should be grateful that I wasn't the sole bread-winner with a family to support, but in my rather emotionally fragile state, I still felt overwhelmed by them. How was I ever going to support myself, cover the bills and pay off the debts accrued from the disastrous investments I'd made in the past? Although I knew I could always turn to her, I hated asking my mother for handouts. Besides, she had repeatedly told me that, rather than persist with the dancing and shows, I should get myself 'a nice little job locally'. But who would employ me when I couldn't sit or stand for any length of time, could barely walk, and sometimes had difficulty even lifting a knife and fork or gripping a pen?

I have always been someone who trusts that things are going to work out somehow. But before the diagnosis, I was so worn out that it was hard to stay positive. I felt helpless because I didn't know what was wrong with me. Now I felt a sense of relief. After a particularly dark, menacing storm, the sun had finally come out again. As with the cancer, once I knew what I was dealing with, I could see a way forward.

In contrast to my grandmother's case, my RA had been caught early and, I was assured, being treated and managed very effectively. As Professor Callan said, things had moved on from when she was a medical student and so many sufferers became wheelchair-bound. She was confident that I would be able to dance again before too long. And happily, she was right!

Now that my RA was being treated, I decided to address those aspects of my life that I'd tended to avoid thinking about – in particular, my personal finances. With the help of Macmillan and my ever-supportive GP I managed to get Employment Seekers Allowance to tide me over. It was backdated too, which was a big help. I had been too proud to ask for it before. Then I confided in my brother about my financial worries, not because I wanted him to do anything but just so I could share the burden. He was surprised but very understanding. I also took independent financial advice from my father's old bank manager, a man I knew I could trust. He was completely non-judgmental and offered me practical advice that made perfect sense. Why had it had taken me so long to do something so obvious? Maybe I'm just a particularly slow learner? Or maybe I was just unwilling to accept that I needed help?

Looking back, it's obvious that I haven't always made the wisest decisions! But then, who has? I've been very lucky in that I've always had the love and support of family and friends. And I wouldn't be the person I am today without these trials and tribulations. At the very least they've made me resilient and more capable of bouncing back from adversity than I ever would have expected – like a 'weeble', the toy that 'wobbles but doesn't fall down' (an analogy that will probably make no sense whatsoever to those under 40 but may conjure up fond childhood memories for older readers).

And of course there's my dancing. Even at my worst, when I was in constant pain and could hardly walk, belly dance was never far from my thoughts. I used to find a flute *taxsim*, close my eyes, and imagine myself bathed in warm sunshine, feeling sand between my toes as my body gently swayed like a reed in the breeze. In my mind – if not in reality – I would undulate to the music, taking my arms above my head in sweeping arabesques, shimmying my shoulders, and tracing smooth circles and figure eights with my hips. And just by doing that I would feel a sense of release; the stiffness would ease, the anxiety and frustration would ebb away, and my spirits would lift. My poor battered body felt loved again. And so, while the NHS provided me with the best possible medical treatment, belly dancing once again proved to be the best medicine for the soul.

Over the years, I've spent hours and hours in hospitals, being bombarded with information, data, test results, words and more words. I have tended to analyse, re-analyse and analyse again what's been said to me, what it actually means, why one word was used rather than another. Sometimes my head has been ready to explode. Dancing has always got me out of my head, and back into my body. When I'm dancing, the jumble of words in my head disappear and I let go completely. I'm a little girl again, dressing up, twirling and spinning around my bedroom, lost in the moment, happy and carefree. And in addition to being the ultimate soul food, dancing is also legal and doesn't result in a hangover.

Yes, as far as I'm concerned, the future's bright, and the future's most definitely sequined!

Chapter 8

Ten Lessons I've Learned (The Hard Way!)

Now I have just turned 50, and in spite of everything, I am happier and more fulfilled than I was at the age of 31. I may have lost my breasts but I've also lost my inhibitions. I enjoy life to the full, cherish my family and friends, and am really grateful for what I've got. I have many friends who haven't made it, so I'm one of the lucky ones. It's true that my life has been more challenging than my younger self would have hoped – more a hike along an overgrown dirt track in the forest than a leisurely walk in the meadows – but it's certainly never been dull. And there have been many clearings in that forest, offering unexpected delights.

I don't profess to have any answers to the meaning of life, but these are the 10 most valuable lessons I've learned from my experiences. I'm sharing them in the hope that they might resonate with you too.

1. To accept myself as I am

I have always been super self-critical. I was never pretty, thin, intelligent, talented or attractive enough for my liking. I always thought everyone was better than me. I was terrified of failure and spent so much time trying to avoid it at all costs, for years pushing myself to be the best I could, to excel in all the different spheres of my life. It was exhausting! But age and life experience have taught me to accept myself just as I am, and in fact, I feel better in my skin now than I did 20 years ago.

2. To practise compassion

Life can be tough but being kind to each other can make the world of difference. There's nothing like being ill and vulnerable to make you value a kind or thoughtful word or deed. When I first had RA I was barely able to walk, and for the first time I fully appreciated the difficulties that many disabled or elderly people face on a daily basis. It made me more thoughtful and understanding, and, I hope, a kinder person.

And, as importantly, I've finally recognised the importance of being kind to *myself*. Just as you are told on a flight to put on your own oxygen mask before attending to those next to you, you need to look after yourself in order to be in a position to help others. After years of beating myself up, I've finally learned to listen to my body, to take time out when

I need it to nurture and nourish myself, and – hardest of all for me – to say 'no' to other people when I need to. And when you're managing chronic conditions such as cancer and RA that's pretty essential.

3. To ask for help when I need it
I don't find it easy to admit when I'm vulnerable and need help. I'd far rather be the one helping others. But I've finally accepted that we all need help sometimes, and, in my experience, other people are very willing to offer it if you'll only let them. In fact, I've found that they love being given the opportunity, and my belly dancing buddies in particular have always risen to the challenge. One caveat – make sure you follow point 4 when it comes to choosing whose help you seek!

4. To trust my instincts
When you're ill, everyone has got advice for you – most of it well-meaning, but not all of it particularly helpful. As I've said, I've learned that it's good to let people help you, but also to recognise when their words and deeds really *aren't* what you need. Cancer is such an emotive word that often it brings out people's worst anxieties, which they can easily project onto you. There are also self-styled 'gurus' who spend their lives telling you how to live yours. At one time I was such a self-help 'junkie', seeking answers in every therapy I came across, that I barely

had time to breathe. Trusting my own instincts and not falling into the trap of believing everything I'm told by others, has become an essential part of being kind to myself.

5. To count my blessings

There are and will always be people worse off than me. I only have to turn on the television, open a newspaper or talk to friends to realise that. I find it helpful to be grateful for what I've got and not to dwell on what I'm lacking. That's not to say that I advocate the adoption of a positive attitude at all costs. Life isn't 'fair' and I think you have to acknowledge all the bad times, the negative emotions, the disappointments and the sorrows before you can move on from them. But wallowing in them has certainly never made me feel any better, while counting my blessings certainly has.

6. To let go of anger and resentment

Now this is a tough one. There are some people I've encountered in my life whose actions have caused me immense pain and hardship – mentally, financially and emotionally. It would be easy to bear grudges and spend hours brooding and plotting my revenge. But it wouldn't change the situation and I'd just be perpetrating more negativity. And, as importantly, it's a waste of valuable energy.

7. To take responsibility for my own wellbeing
Doctors don't know everything. How can they? But it's easy to feel completely at their mercy when you're going through a major illness, and feeling particularly vulnerable. And, sadly, there are too many who continue to treat patients as a medical condition rather than a person. I've always found it helpful to consider myself as team leader and regard all the doctors, consultants, oncologists, nurses *et al* as part of my team, experts whom I can call upon to give me their specialist advice. Ultimately, though, I'm in charge.

Besides, your physical health is only one aspect of your total wellbeing. Your emotional, physical and mental states are every bit as important. Again, what works for one person doesn't for another; you need to find your own route to good health and happiness.

8. To slow down
Being ill forces you to move at a completely different pace. I look back at the amount I used to cram into a single day and it makes me want to lie down! I really don't know how I managed it. But I did, until my body protested and forced me to stop. And while I was doing so much I never fully appreciated any of it; I was always focusing on the next task, the next deadline. Now I do much less, I have the time to fully appreciate and enjoy my life.

9. To laugh, play and be silly

I like to think that I have a well-developed laughter muscle. But I've learned that it needs exercising regularly or you can lose the habit. And where cancer is concerned people around you tend to be so serious. Studies have shown that while children laugh 300–400 times a day, adults barely make it past 10. My belly dance buddies have always brought out my playful and silly side. By not taking myself too seriously and seeing the funny side of whatever life throws at me, I've coped better and kept (relatively) sane. Besides, laughter costs nothing, releases endorphins and de-stresses, and is utterly infectious – in the best possible way!

10. To follow my heart

I believe that we are all on our own path. People come in and out of our lives and join us for some of the way, but ultimately we're on our own. I've learned that it serves no purpose to compare myself with others and want what they have, or to pursue someone else's dreams. Sadly, it took three incidences of cancer for me to take the plunge and follow my heart. So, I urge you, don't wait for illness or trauma to pursue your passion, whatever it may be. Throw caution to the wind and dig out those dancing shoes! Being alive is wonderful, but it isn't enough. You have to do what brings you alive. And for me, that was and is belly dancing.

Further Information

Cancer Support and Information
These two organisations offer invaluable support if
you are affected by cancer in any way:

www.macmillan.org.uk
www.mariecurie.org.uk

This is a great charity doing research into cancer,
which relies on donations to continue its work:

www.cancerresearchuk.org

The Royal Marsden Hospital, which has kept me
fit and well over the last 18 years, is pioneering new
treatments and techniques to save lives, but needs
financial support to do so:

www.royalmarsden.org

The following charities offer amazing help and support to people specifically with breast cancer:

www.breastcancercare.org.uk
www.breakthrough.org.uk
www.cancerkin.org.uk
www.thehaven.org.uk
www.maggiescentres.org

This UK-registered charity is aimed at promoting awareness, early detection, treatment and after-care of breast cancer for women in Egypt:

www.justbecause.org.uk

Support with Rheumatoid Arthritis
For information about rheumatoid arthritis, what it is, how it can be managed and living with the condition:

www.nras.org.uk

All Things Belly Dance
The JWAAD Book of Belly Dance is a gorgeous, fully illustrated book that covers all the basic belly dance moves, different dance styles, Middle Eastern music rhythms, costuming and background information. For full details of this and a range of belly dance activities and training:

www.jwaad.com

For belly dance classes in your area:

www.thejta.org

Sequins on My Balcony
I would like to acknowledge the contribution of
everyone who has helped me to create and develop
the show, and in particular:

Peta Lily – friend, co-writer and director:
www.petalily.com

Anne Mayer, Cec, Cleo and everyone at the
Rosemary Branch Theatre:
www.rosemarybranch.co.uk

Do Get in Touch!
Join my mailing list to find about future shows,
events and activities, plus Dance Yourself Happy,
Creative Dancer and Belly Dance classes and
workshops: yvette_cowles@yahoo.co.uk

Like on Facebook: Sequins on My Balcony
Follow on Twitter: @YvetteCowles
www.DanceYourselfHappy.com

Moving Memoirs

Stories of hope, courage and the power of love…

If you loved this book, then you will love our Moving Memoirs eNewsletter

Sign up to…

- Be the first to hear about new books

- Get sneak previews from your favourite authors

- Read exclusive interviews

- Be entered into our monthly prize draw to win one of our latest releases before it's even hit the shops!

Sign up at

www.moving-memoirs.com

Harper True.
Time to be inspired

Write for us

Do you have a true life story of your own?

Whether you think it will inspire us, move us, make us laugh or make us cry, we want to hear from you.

To find out more, visit

www.harpertrue.com or send your ideas to harpertrue@harpercollins.co.uk and soon you could be a published author.